P9-BYZ-500

D0002777

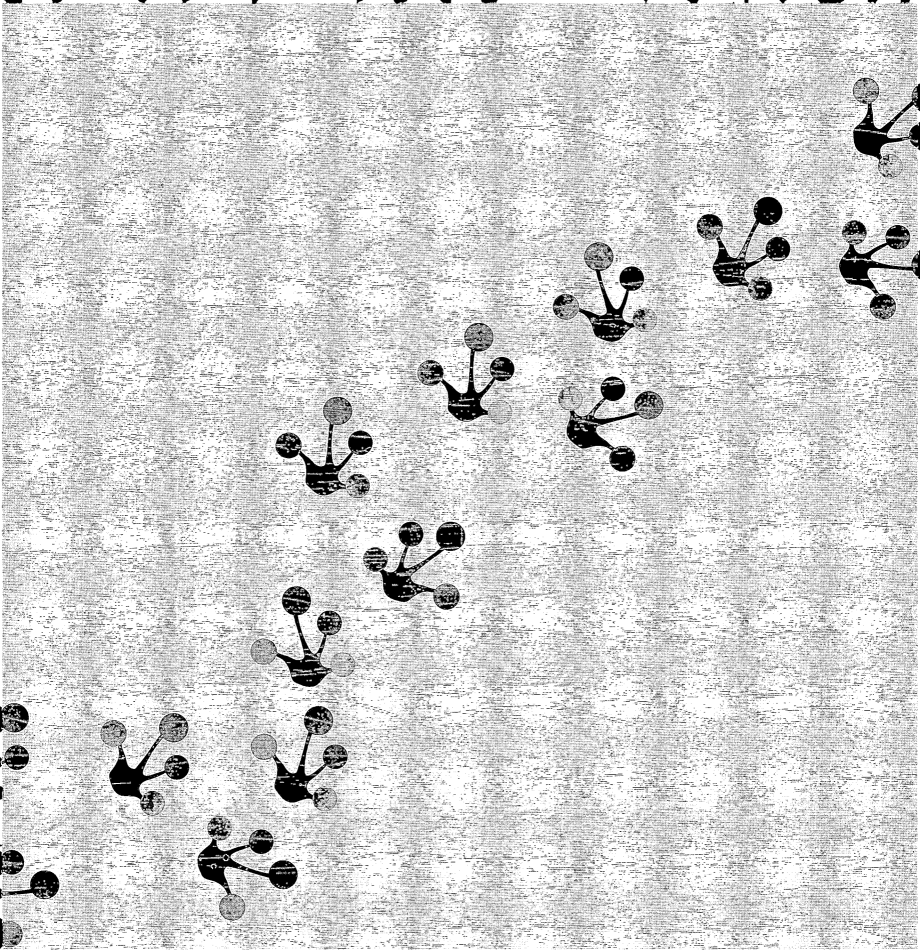

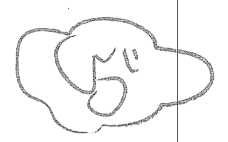

To my birth parents who gave me the gift of family.

And to my family ... Mom, Dad and my brother, Jim.
Thank you for loving me long before you met me,
and especially after you really got to know me.

Gratitude (n.) grat·i·tude. An extremely positive emotion of thankfulness that bursts from Jillian's heart and is dedicated toward the following people whom helped bring this book to life and helped Jillian find a happy ending to one of her fairytales:

My dollzers Craig, my little cutie-patooties Max and Hayden, this baby in my belly who I can't wait to cuddle, Mom, Dad, Jim, Cathy, Ryan, Timmy, G-ma Z, Gerrie (Mrs. M), my rock in business Kelly, the amazingly talented Erin, the artistic and patient Maria, Kristen, Molly, Michael, Renee, Jessica, Kerry, my loving extended family (I am Irish Catholic, so if I named them all it would take more than a page) and to all my incredibly fun and encouraging friends that I have met on my life's journey.

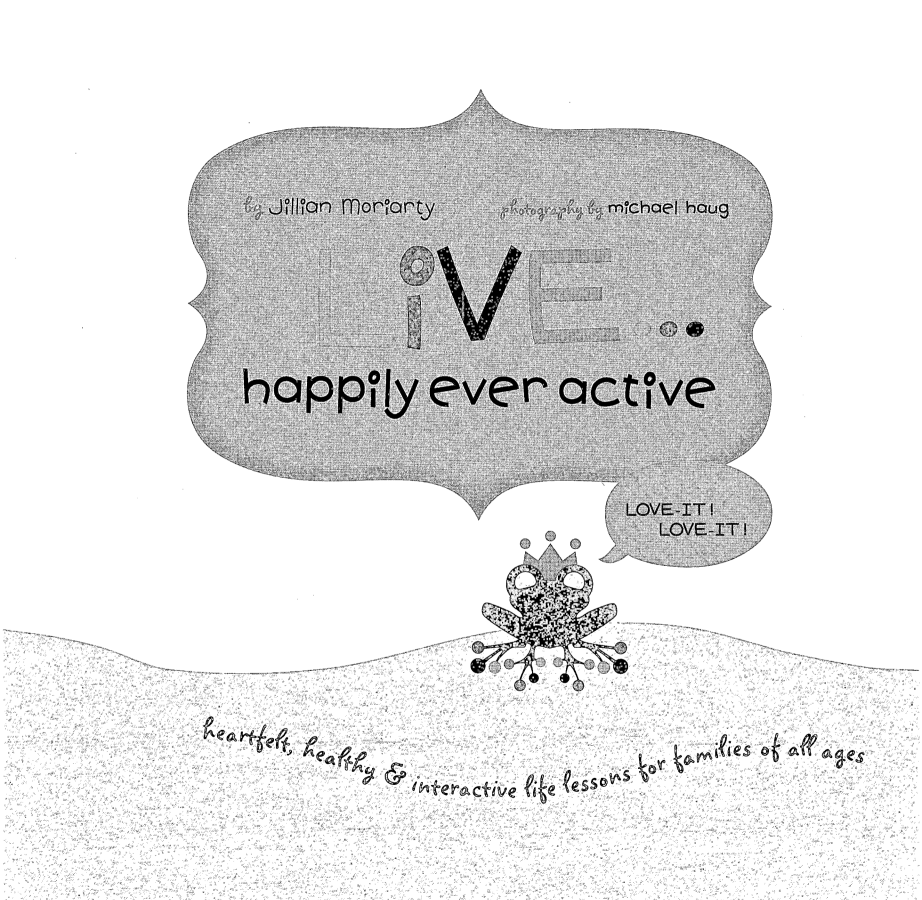

by Jillian Moriarty   photography by michael haug

LiVE...

happily ever active

LOVE-IT!
LOVE-IT!

heartfelt, healthy & interactive life lessons for families of all ages

Bringing back the WE and the Wheee in family!

It's the 21st century and the quintessential family is no longer June, Ward, Wally and "the Beav." Today, families come in all different sizes and shapes, blends of color and ethnicity, and mixes of genetics or even no biological heritage at all. What is common to all families, however, is the big L-word. Can you guess which word I am thinking of? Yes, it is **LOVE!**

Also, with text-messages, e-mail, apps and downloads, families do not communicate or move as they used to... or as well as they should. I believe families need to touch and be touched, not just be "in touch." What happened to laughing with one another instead of L-O-L, smiling instead of :), or going on a hike to learn about nature rather than Googling it? Sure everything is right at our fingertips, but families are missing out on making some real connections. That is what inspired us at Happily Ever Active® to create a movement which we term, "the new family fairytale," and this book is an integral part in finding a "happily ever" ending.

This book brings family together to deepen their loving connection with one another through learning and movement exploration. It goes well beyond reading and literacy and enhances the well being of families: body, mind and spirit. This book is for all ages

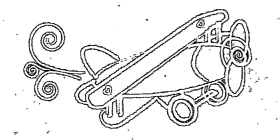

as the life lessons are reminders of health, etiquette, values, and pure goodness everyone needs every day! From adorably big-bellied, drooling babies to wise, wrinkled elders, this short and sweet book makes a big and powerful impact. The lessons empower families with knowledge of yoga, Pilates, traditional fitness, good manners and heart-felt interaction. Families will not only learn together, but learn from one another especially as you *Explore More* (an enhanced version of our book) which details each and every page allowing kids of all ages to stretch and grow their bodies and minds. A sample of our *Explore More* is at the end of this book and available in its full version on our website at www.LiveHappilyEverActive.com.

I hope this book inspires families everywhere to improve their understanding and compassion for each other, to find goodness in themselves and in their surroundings, to better their physical and emotional well-being, and to live happily ever active together. Heck — who doesn't want a piece of this happy pie?!? I'll take two, please!

Our mission to empower, embrace and enrich lives starts with family... with pure love. From this great starting point we hope the whole country, the whole world, will embrace their own family and realize that all of us are part of a bigger family!

Enjoy life's adventure with your family...

My mom tells me:
Life is a journey.

Take one step at a time,

Always bring your body along for the ride.

Pack only what you need,

And leave everything else behind.

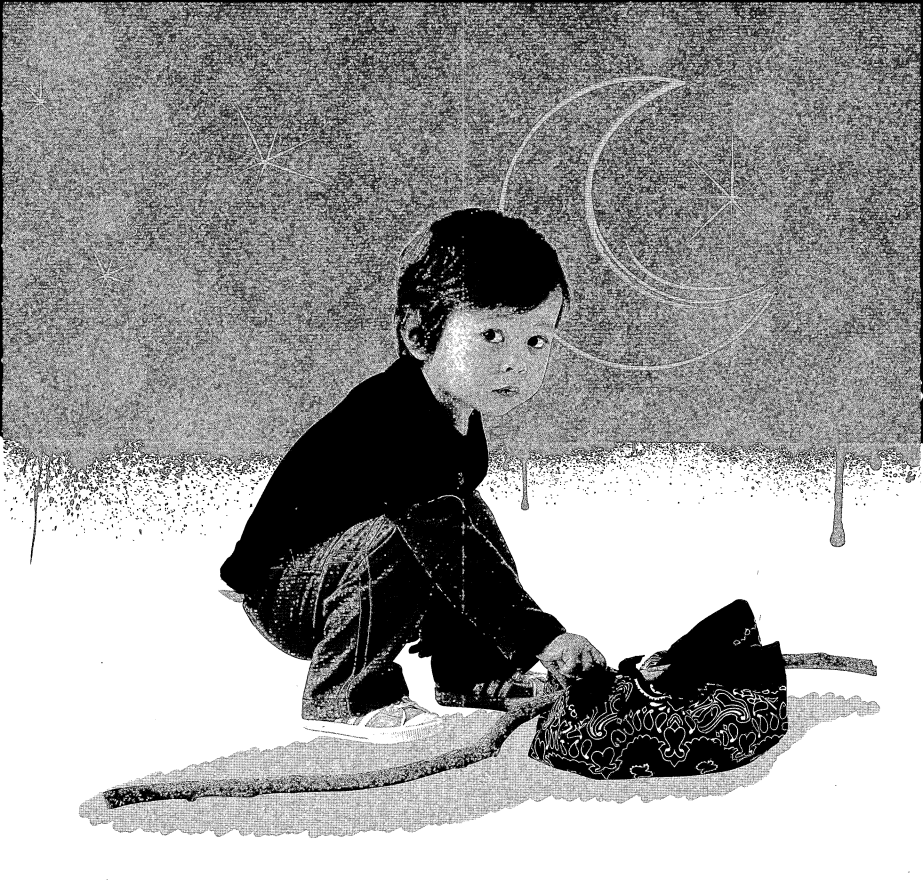

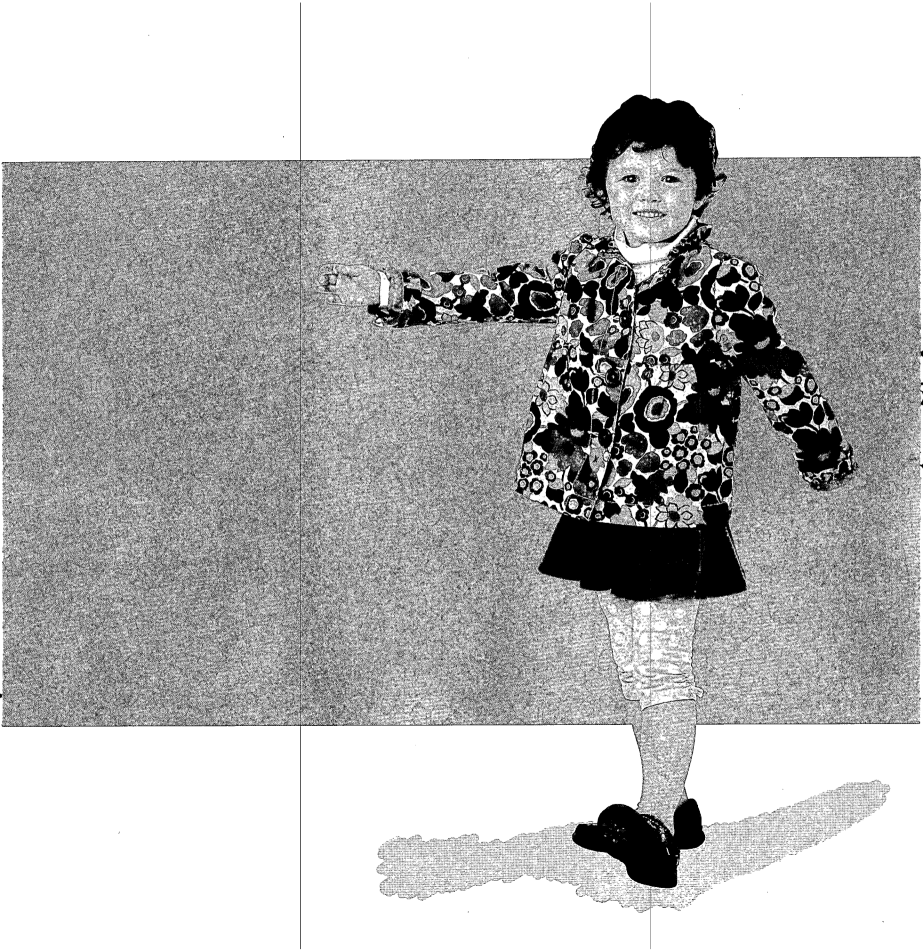

Heel ... Toe. Heel ... toe.

Big 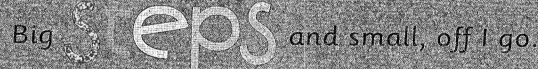 and small, off I go.

Heel ... Toe. Heel ... toe.

Some steps are quick and some are S l o w.

My dad reminds me:
There will be ...

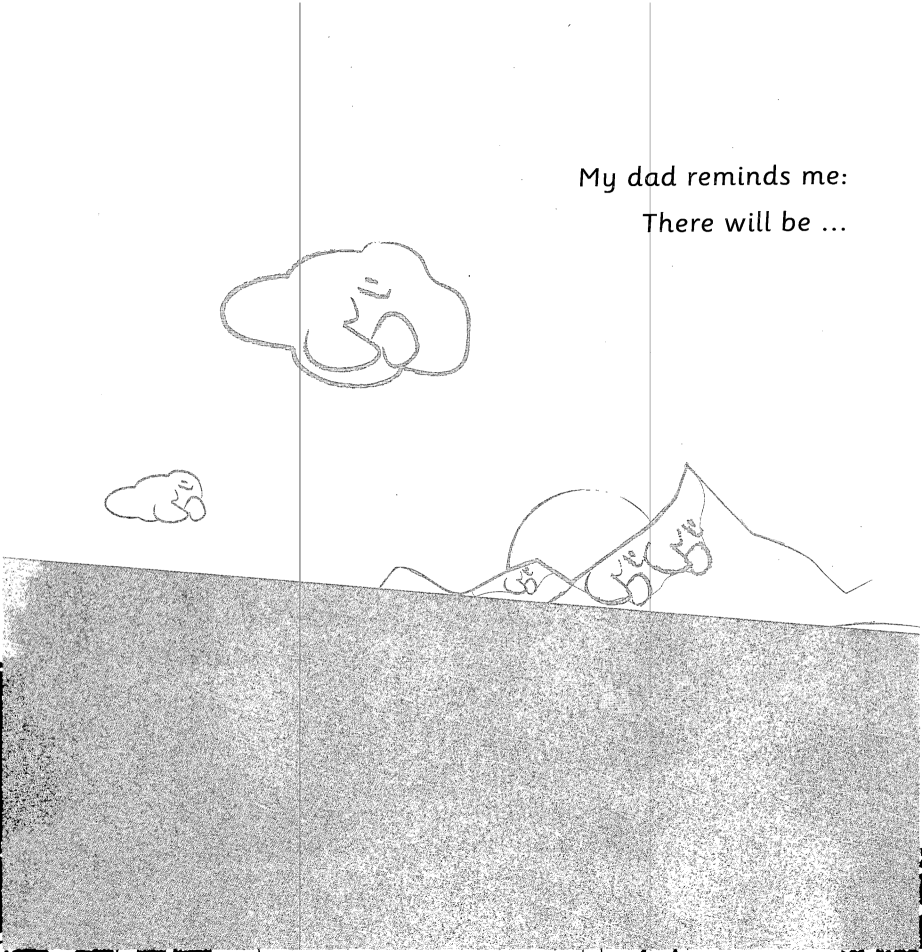

mountains to climb.

One-Two-Three-Four-Five
Six-Seven-Eight-Nine!

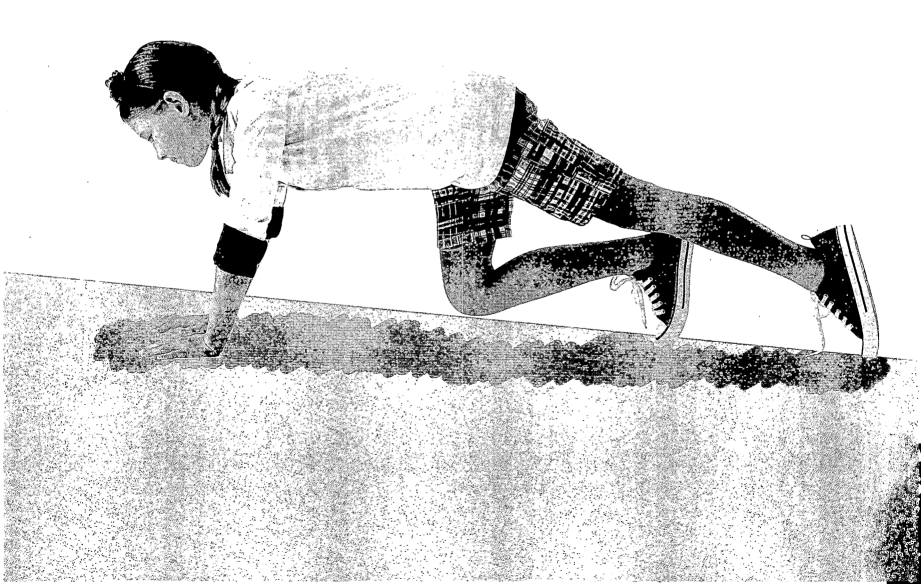

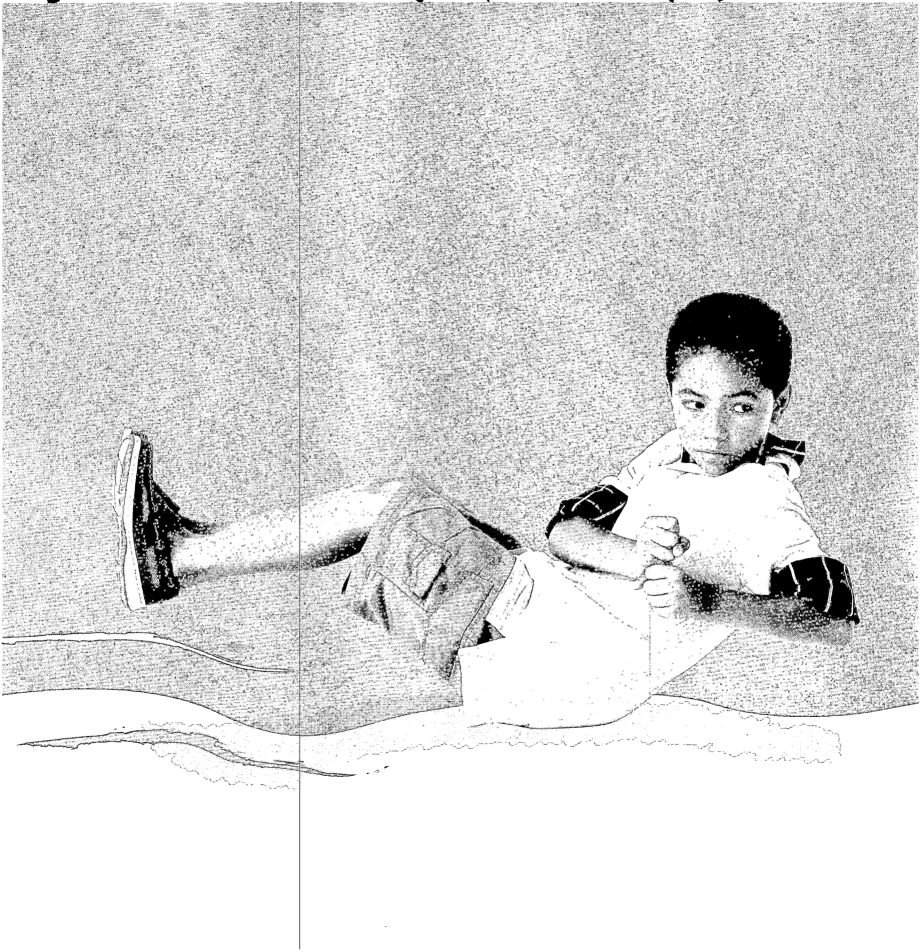

Life is not always smooth sailing,

Bring a 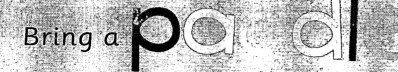paddle,

And everything will be just fine.

My big sister says:

If I feel concern or worry

To take it slow and **breathe.**

Deep Inhales and Exhales.

One ... Two ... & Three,

Will put my mind at ease.

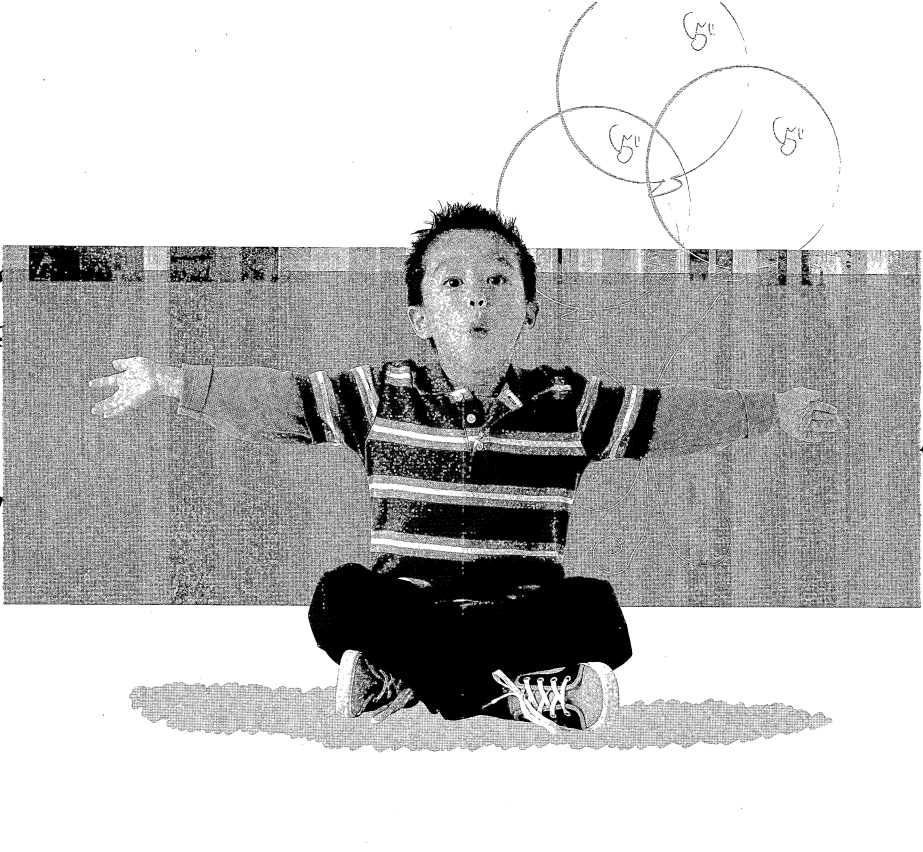

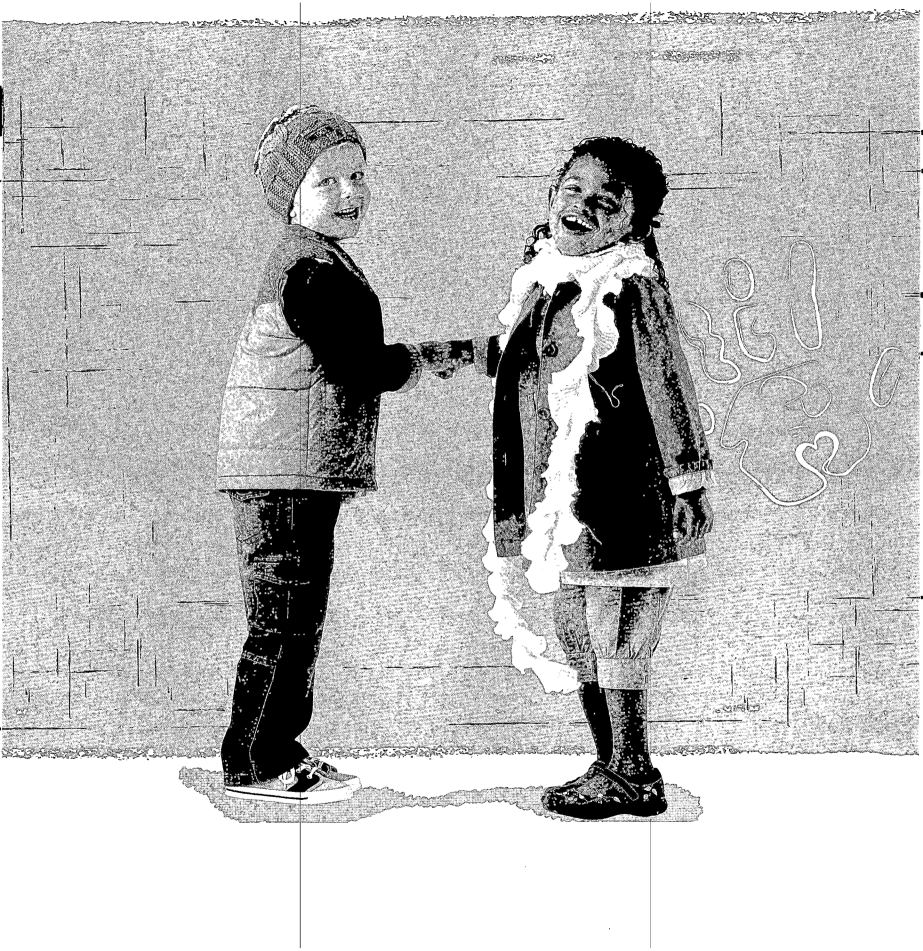

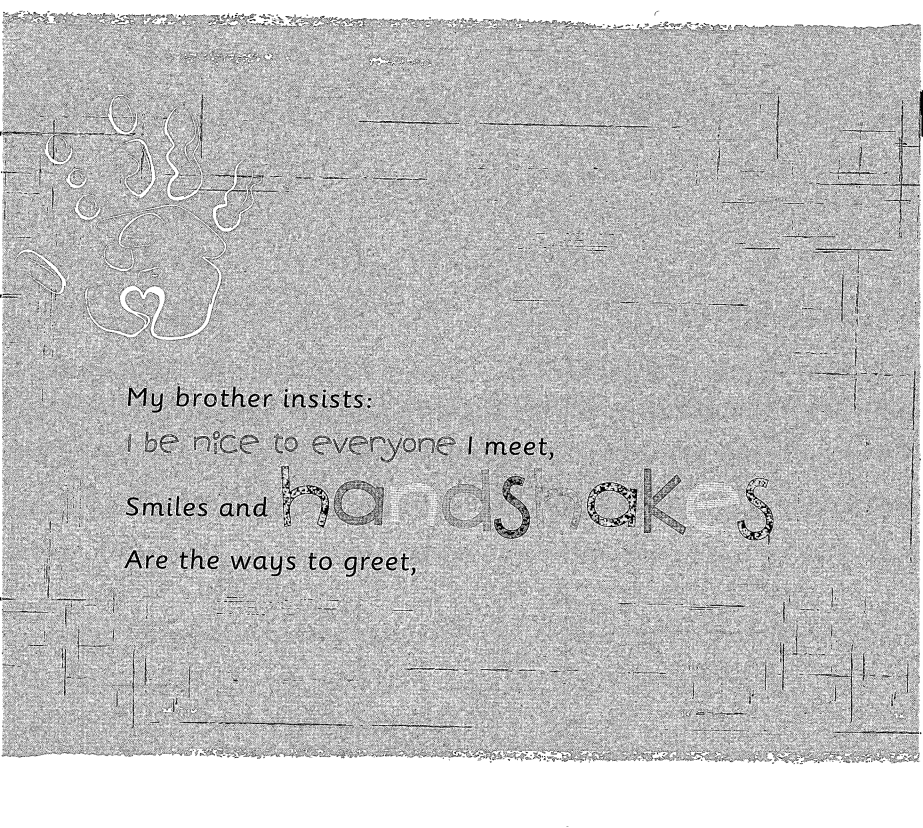

My brother insists:

I be nice to everyone I meet,

Smiles and handshakes

Are the ways to greet,

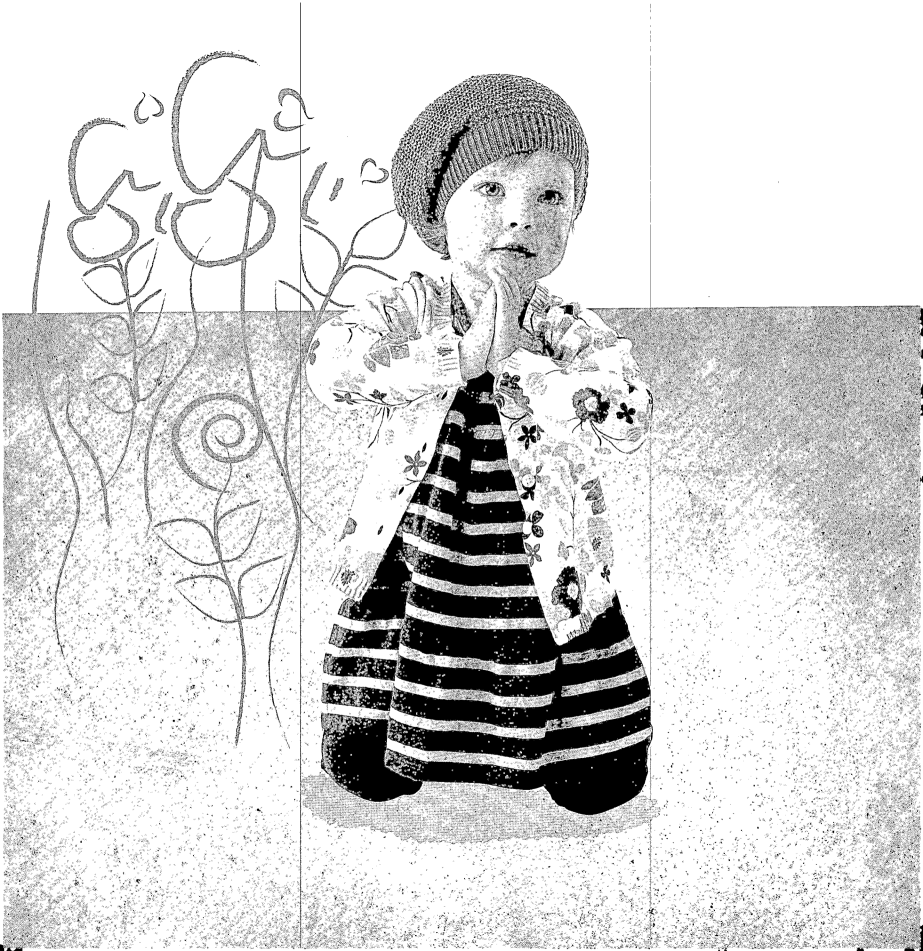

And always remember good manners.
Say thank you and say please.

So with my family's blessings and advice,

I take off on my journey 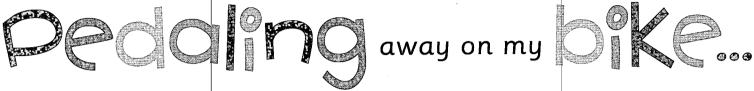 away on my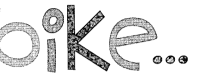

I am so excited, but not in a flurry,

For I remember that momma said

To take my own sweet time and never hurry.

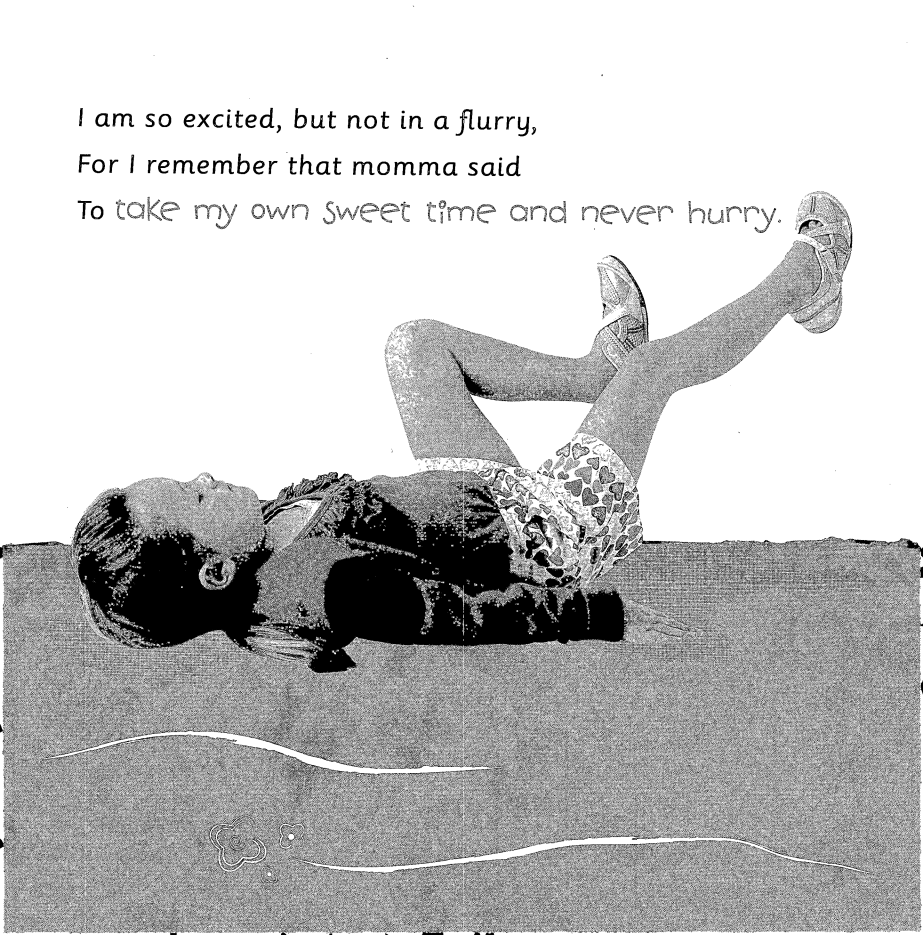

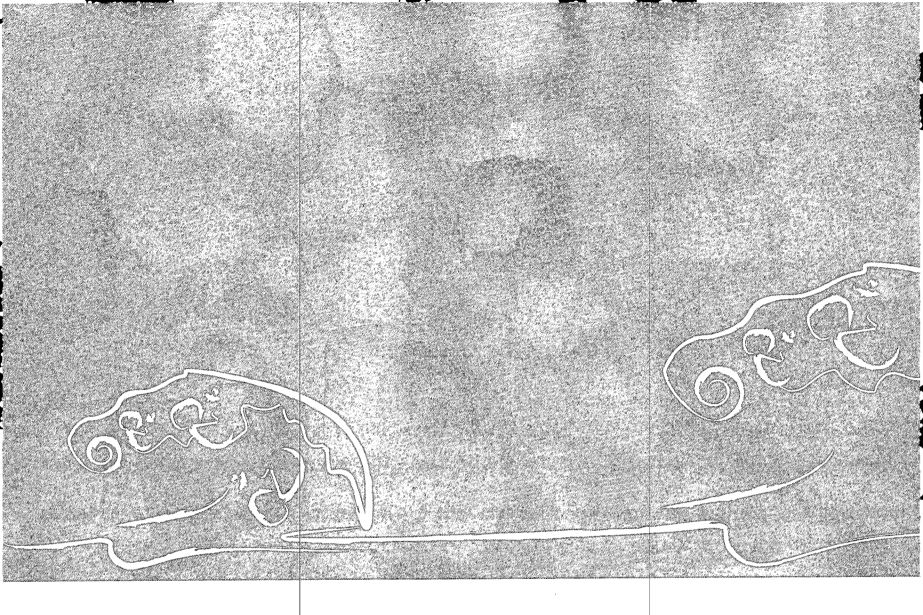

My first stop is the ocean
Where I watch big, frothy, waves

Roooooooll in ... Roooooooll out
Roooooooll in ... Roooooooll out

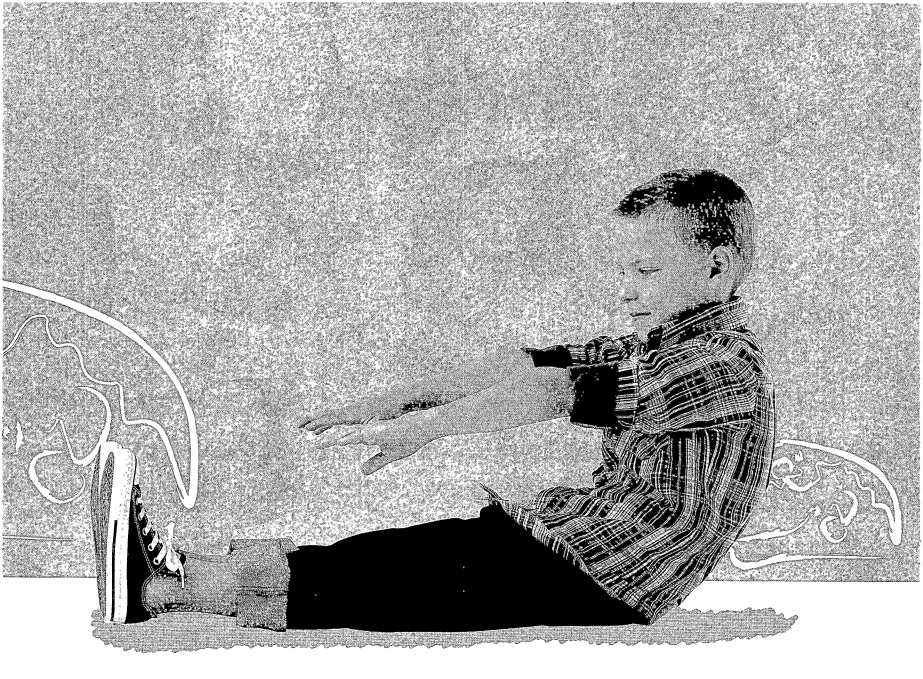

The tide, well, it may change,

But the waves roll in and out

All through night and day.

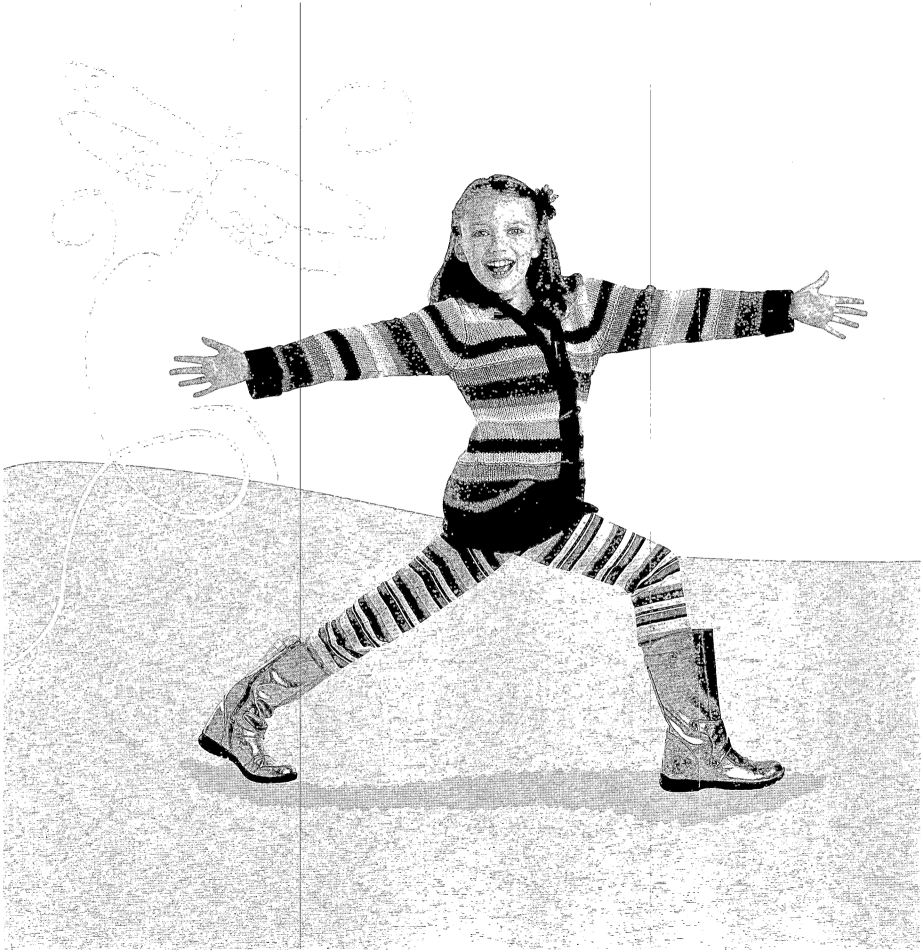

As I continue on my adventure,

A sparkling buzz surrounds me,

Shiny gold and green,

It is a **dragonfly**

Who becomes my company.

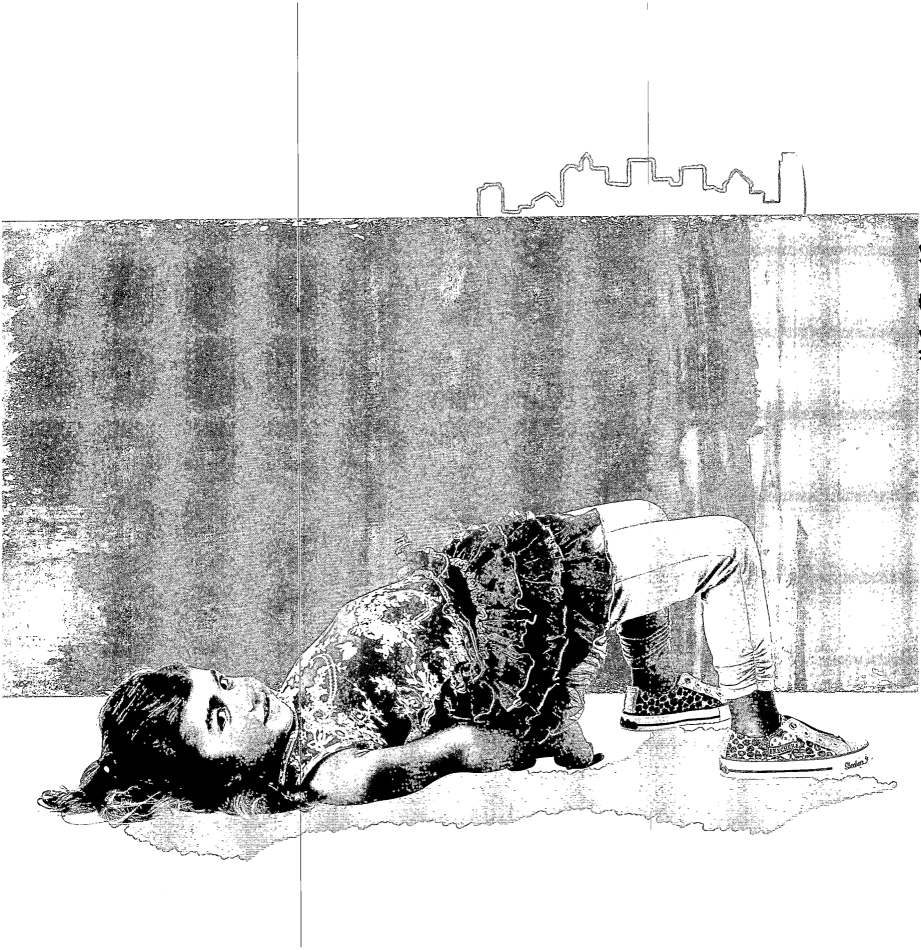

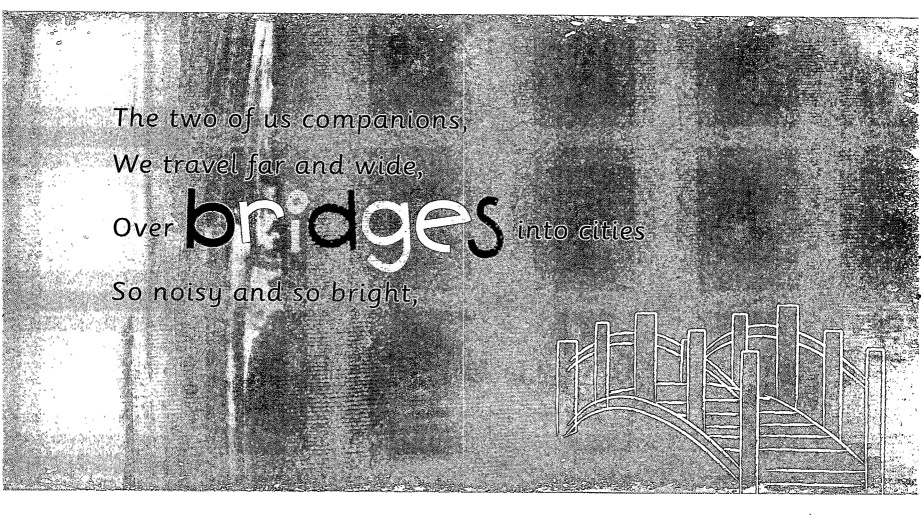

The two of us companions,
We travel far and wide,
Over **bridges** into cities
So noisy and so bright,

Across great, green, grassy fields

Where COWS roam the countryside,

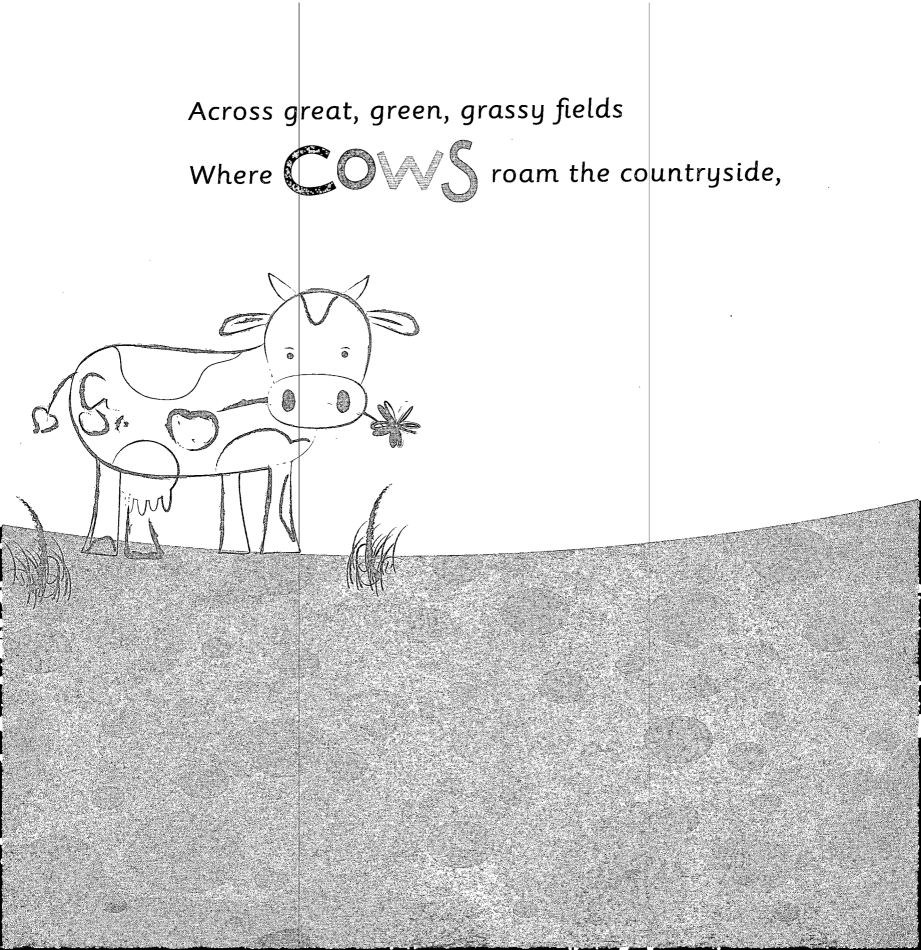

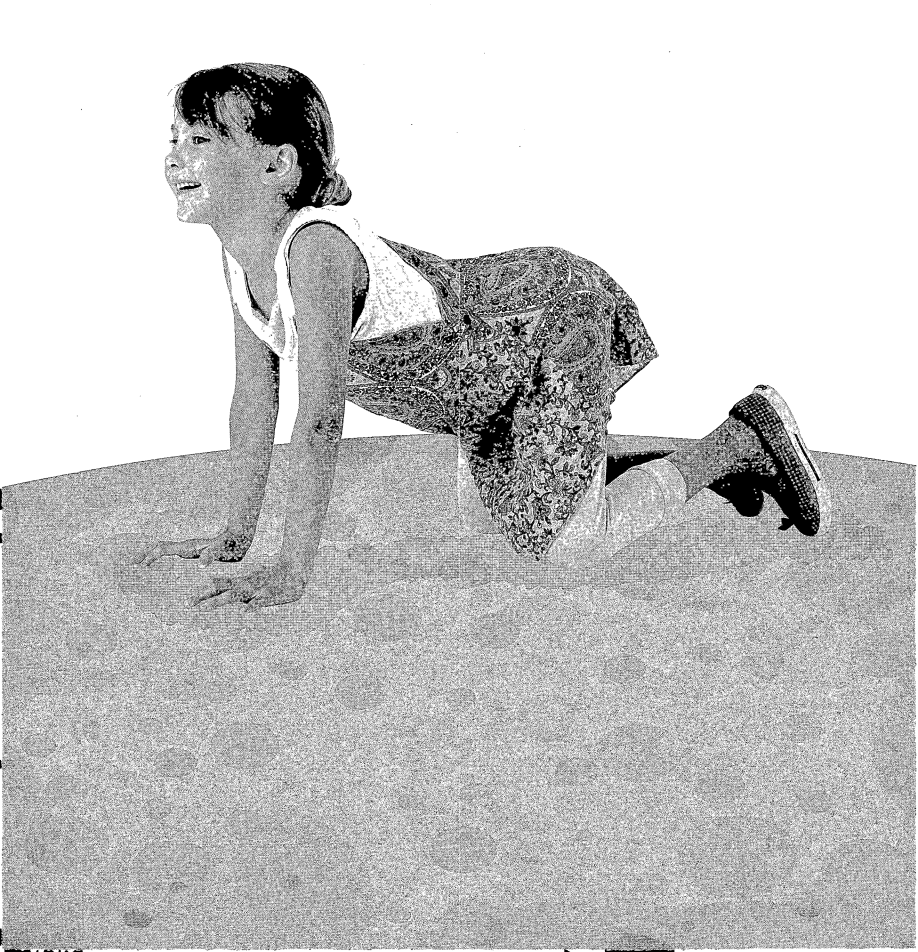

Into forests, dense with trees,
That shade us from the hot sunlight.

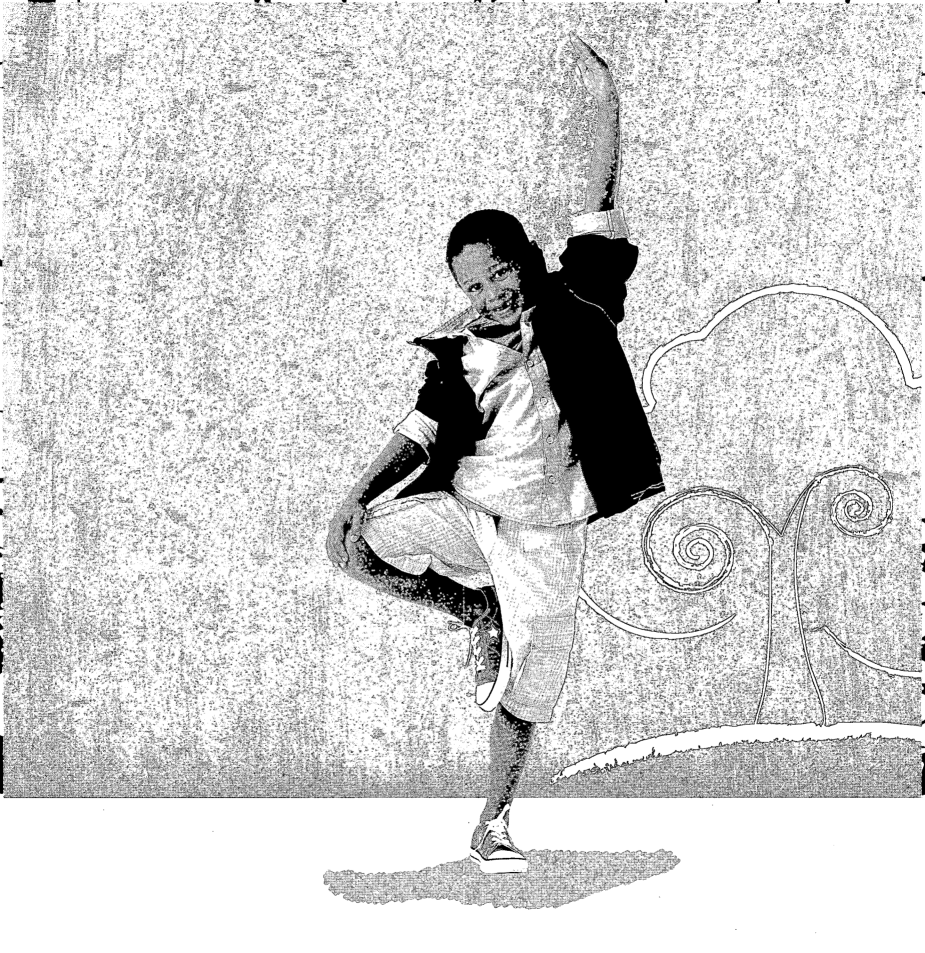

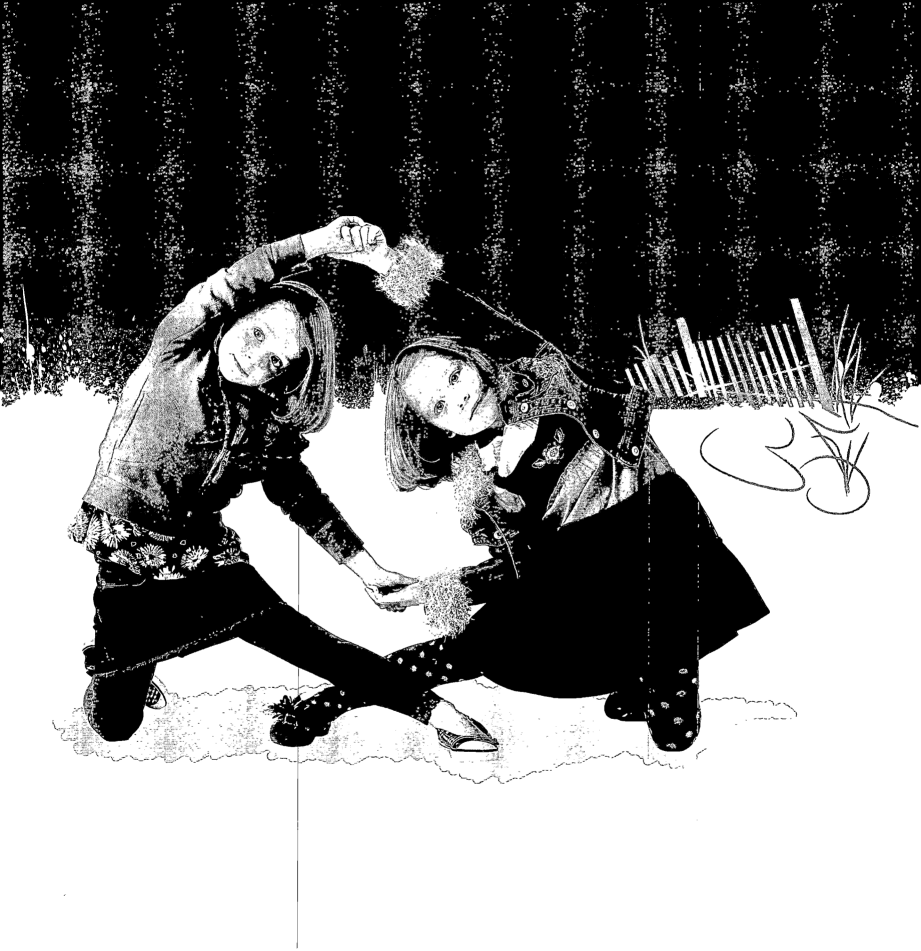

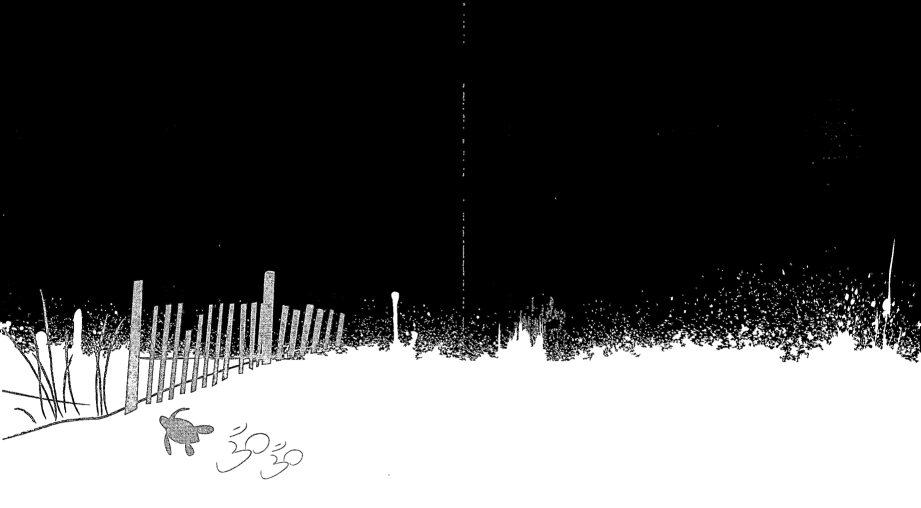

And when the ride gets bumpy,

Or someone's in a jam,

We know we have each other

To lend a **helping hand.**

Trust, respect and honesty,

These things we need to have,

And we can Conquer anything —

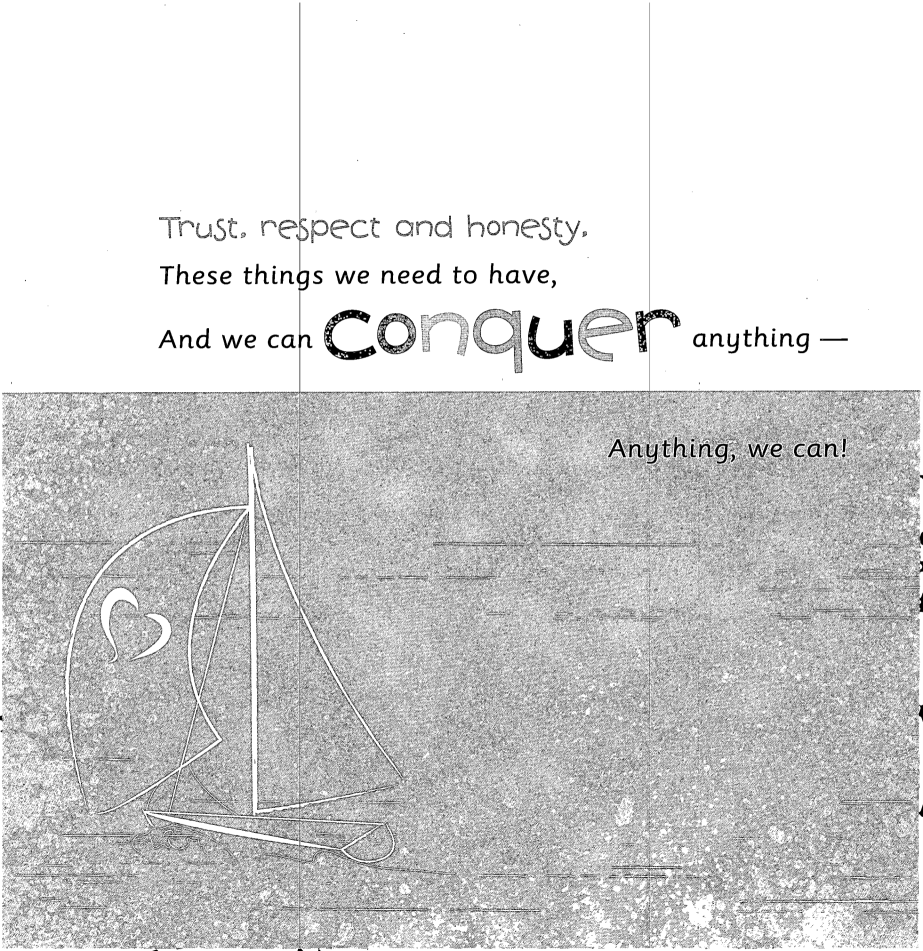

Anything, we can!

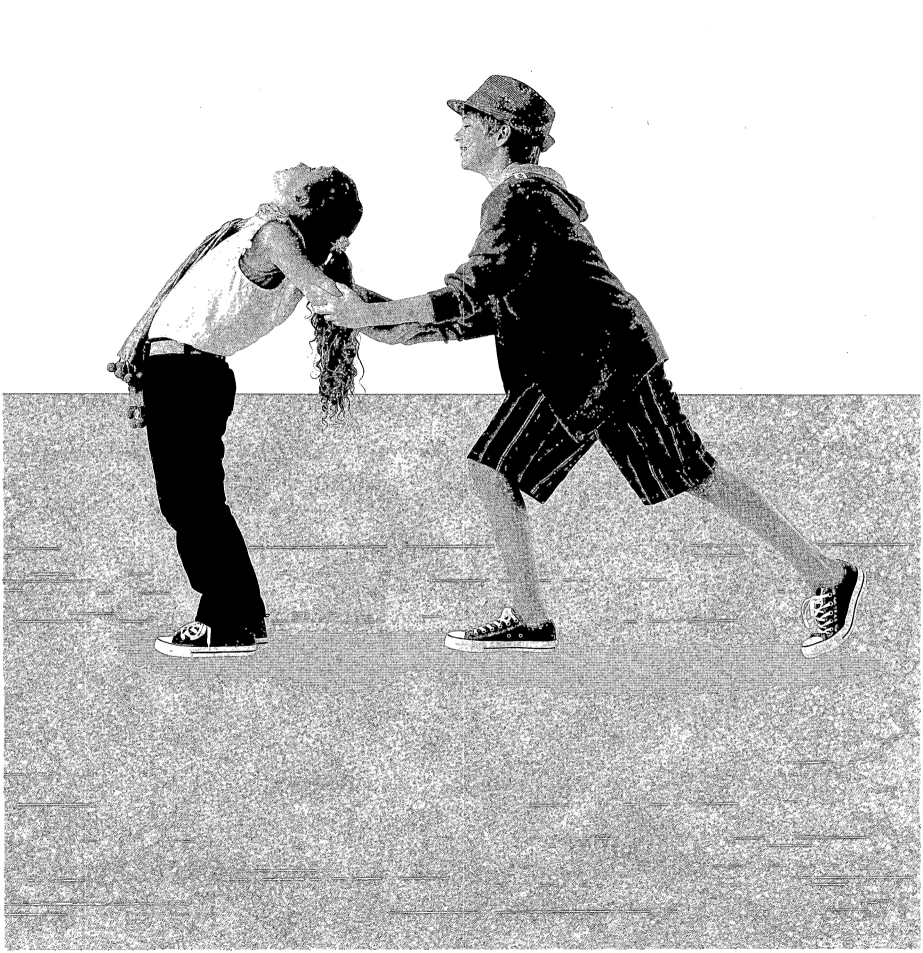

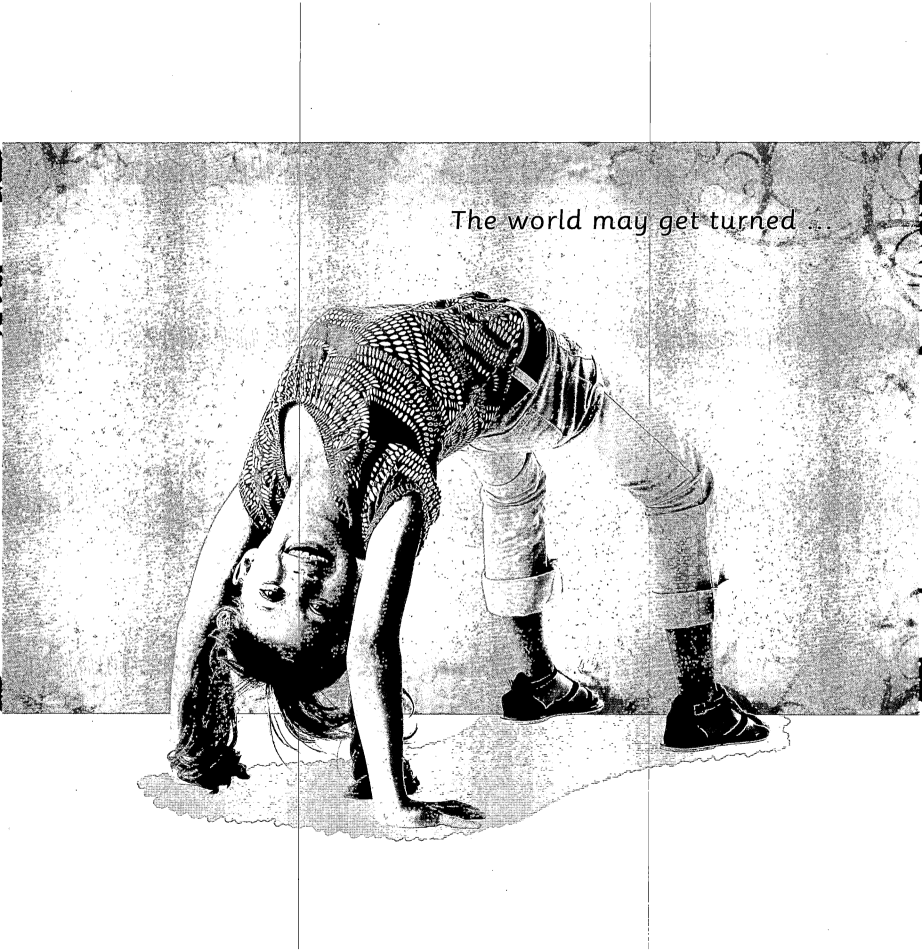

The world may get turned ...

upside down,

But in these crazy times,

I remember Grandpa's wisdom

To smile and not to frown,

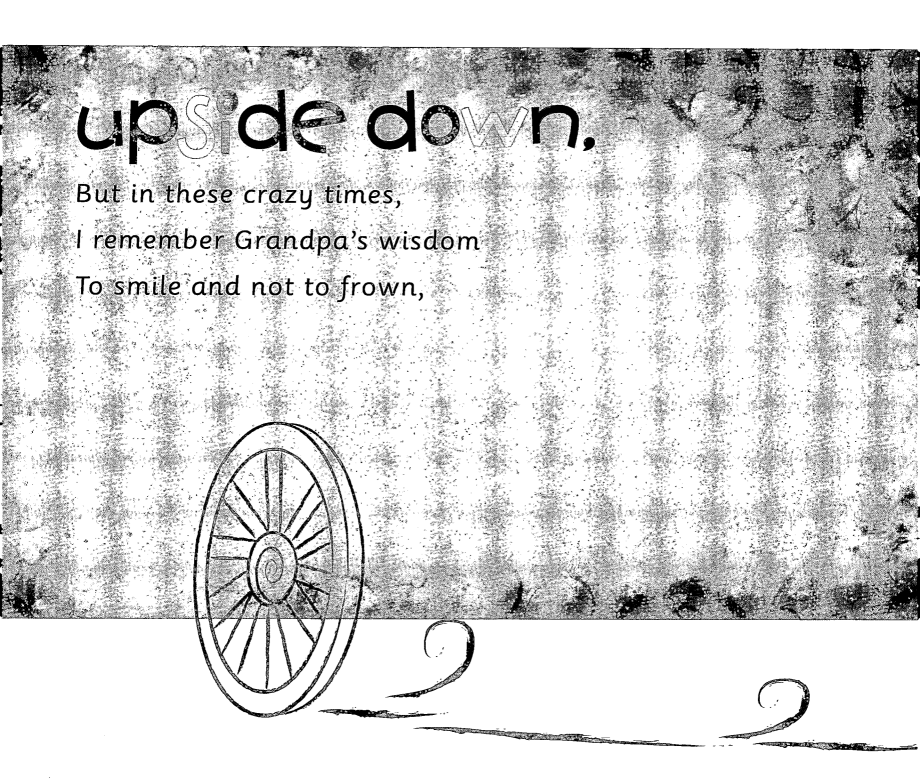

And to find the positive.

Even in a world that is **Spinning**

round and round.

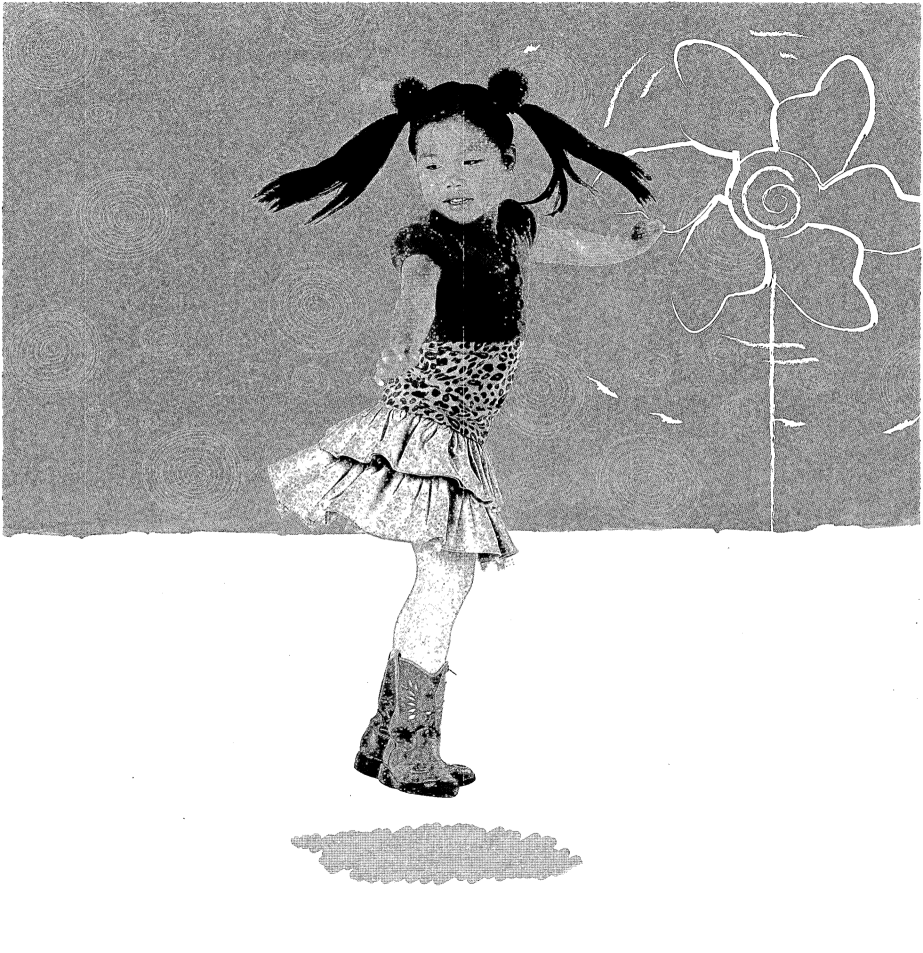

So through these **twists** and turns I travel
And grow stronger every day,
My mind and body connecting
More and more along the way.

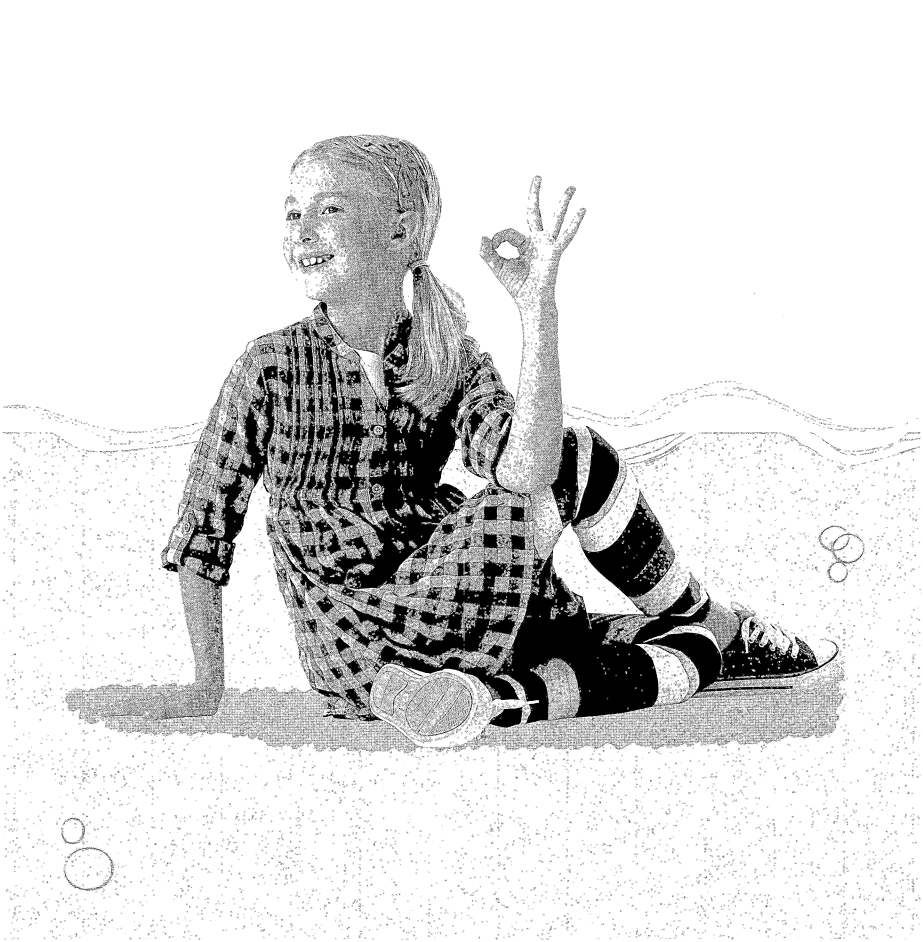

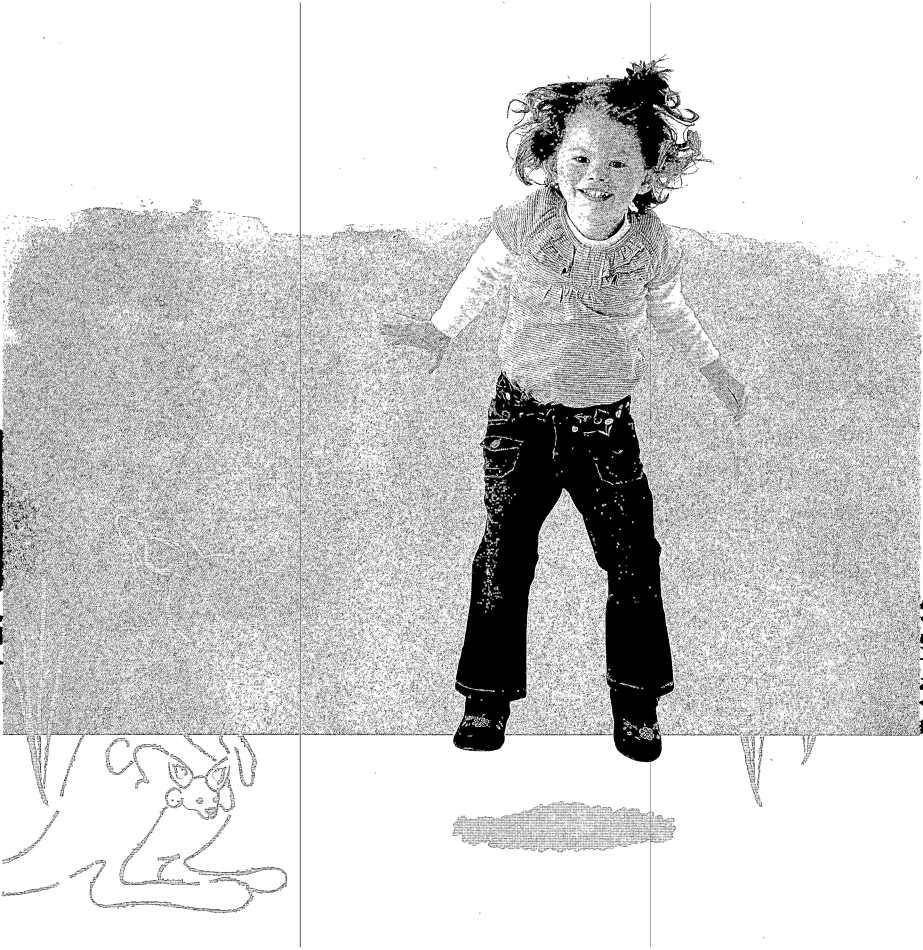

My heart beats happily inside my chest,

My lungs sing out thank you,

For all the running, jumping and exercise

This journey puts me through,

My body cries out:

YIPPEE SKIPPEE and YAHOO!

Throughout life's expedition,
I hear Grandma's voice repeat:

Keep your eyes wide open

And watch carefully,

For there is so much beauty

In this world to see.

Even in the fine, silky web,

A little 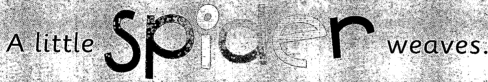spider weaves.

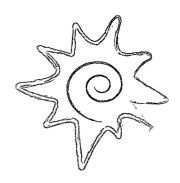

I am proud of all my endeavors,
Making it through thick and thin,

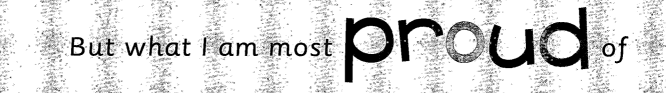

But what I am most **proud** of
Is the person I have found within!

My experiences, my family and their love.

And the friends I meet on my way,

Remind me to ...

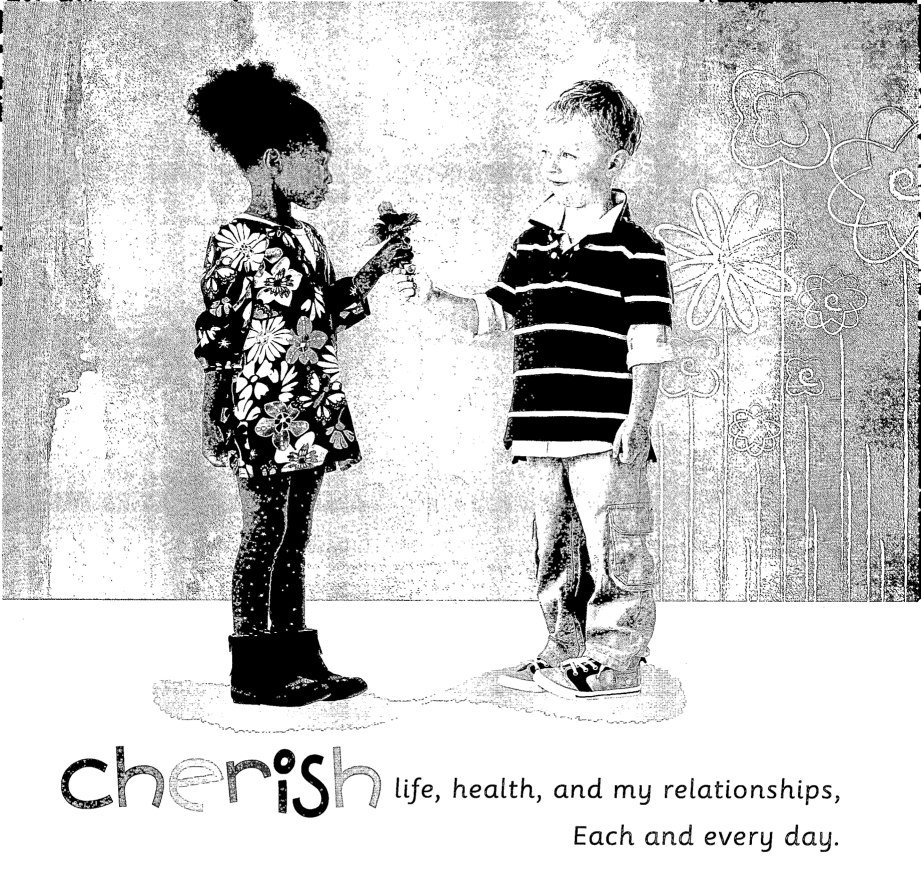

cherish life, health, and my relationships,
Each and every day.

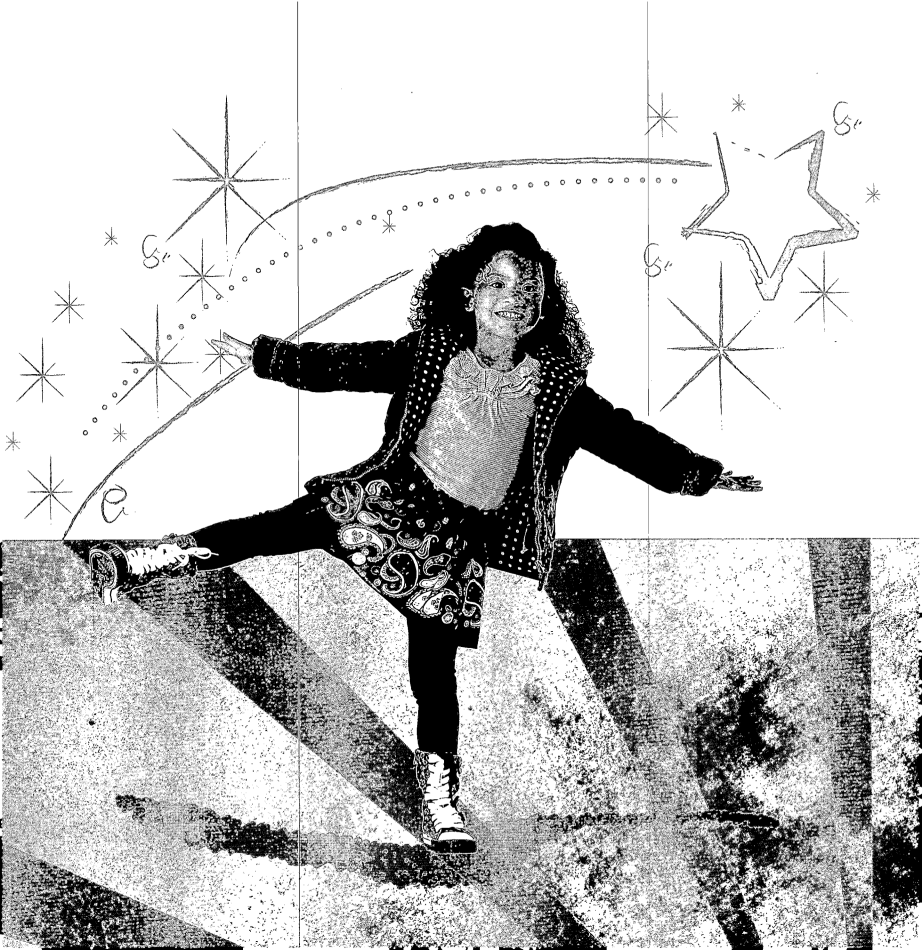

I know I still have much to learn,

For my journey, it persists.

I continue to uncover my spirit, my inner light,

My values, my passions, my dreams,

My true beauty shining bright,

Like a Star twinkling in the night.

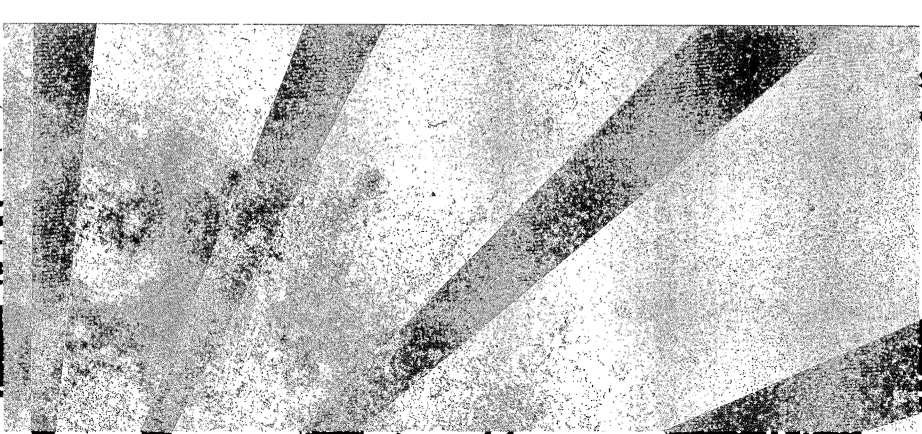

So if I had one piece of advice,

Now, to give to you,

Simply put:

Smile, breathe and enjoy the life you live.

Surround yourself with people you love.

Exercise, eat healthy, always be willing to give,

And you will set off into the sunset

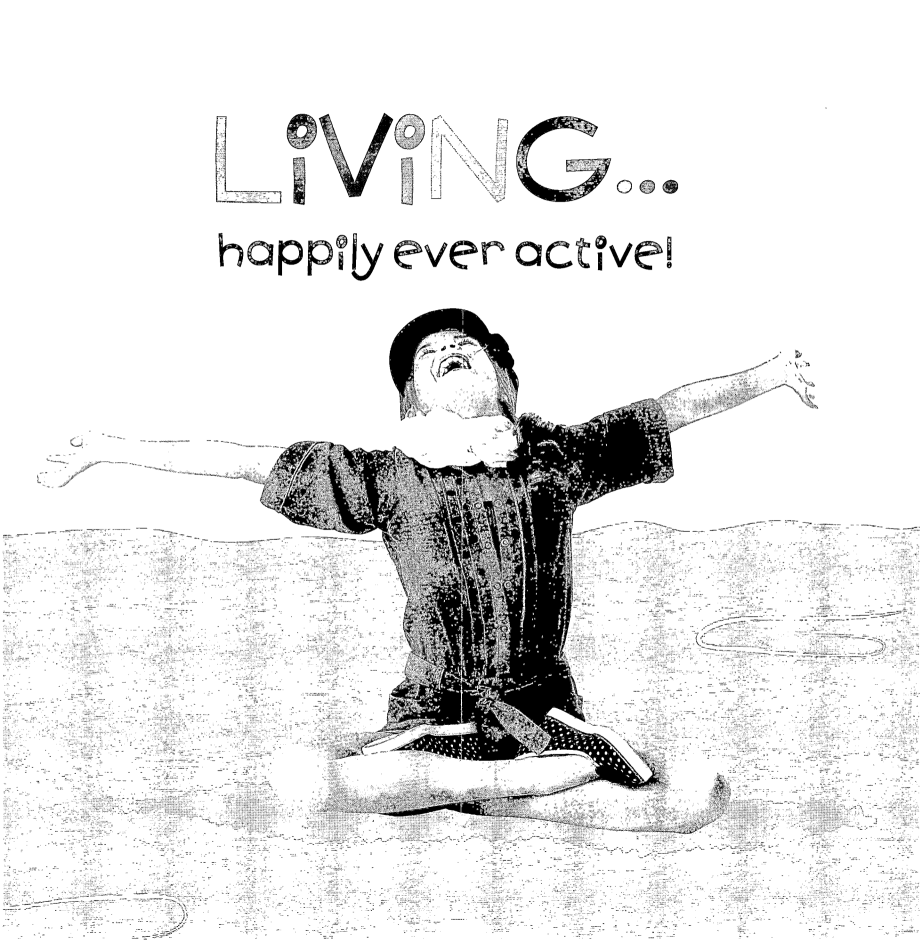

explore more

Take your family trip through life one step further with our *Explore More* manual. This "travel guide" provides more description for each page of this book including instruction on how to perform the yoga & Pilates-based exercises, cues for converting individual activities into full-on family interactivities, thoughtful questions to inspire better communication and understanding of self and each other, fun facts and silly stories to enjoy and more! Explore More is easily downloadable from our website and is sure to make your journey more jubilant. Visit **www.LiveHappilyEverActive.com**.

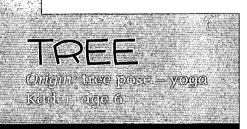

TREE
Origin: tree pose — yoga
Korder — age 6

www.LiveHappilyEverActive.com

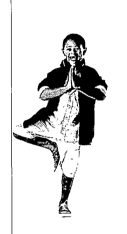

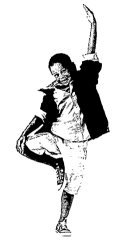

Stand as tall as a Sequoia tree. Lift right foot to place against left inner thigh. (Tisk-tisk! Don't let your foot push into knee joint.) Open hip out wide with knee facing directly to side. Bring your hands to Namaste.

Continue to breathe steady and slow and stay balanced. Grow deep roots through your strong, tree trunk leg and reach up with your long, leafy-branched arms.

Exhale out a strong gust of wind and let your tree sway to the side. Right hand to knee as your torso leans.

Repeat tree standing on other leg.

Practice. Practice. There is no perfect! And if for some reason your tree falls down, there is no reason to frown. Smile and shout TIMBER! on your way to the ground. Then, pick yourself up and try another round.

A little known fact ... The five tallest trees in the world are:
- Coast Redwood (a type of Sequoia) grows to 379 feet! — California, USA
- Australian Mountain-ash — Tasmania, Australia
- Coast Douglas-fir — Oregon, USA
- Sitka Spruce — California, USA
- Giant Sequoia — California, USA

a little something about the creators

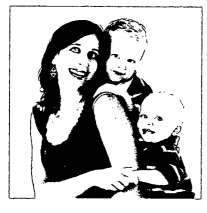

Author & Mommy

Jillian Moriarty, MSPT has over 15 years of experience as a licensed physical therapist, a bodyworker, and a certified yoga and Pilates practitioner. She strives to improve the health and happiness of all of her patients and clients from neonatal intensive care to special needs pediatrics to geriatrics. With this book, her first book for children, she combines her expertise in the health and wellness industry with her passion for putting family first. Jillian motivates families to be active and healthy, learn together and from one another, laugh until they snort, and love out loud.

Jillian and her family, including 160 pound St Bernard "puppy," enjoy tickle-fests, cooking homemade pizzas, exploring the outdoors, and kissing each other good morning, good afternoon and goodnight. They live in Wayzata, MN.

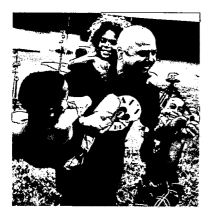

Photographer

Michael Haug has been in the photography business for over a decade. He has a great appreciation for his experiences and career growth as only those who've worked their way up from the bottom know. He is a gregarious guy known for dancing on set to get kids to laugh and smile. He executes even the toughest jobs with patience and humor. www.MichaelHaug.com

www.LiveHappilyEverActive.com

Library of Congress Catalog Number: 2010936765
ISBN 10: 1-935204-27-0
ISBN 13: 978-1-935204-27-5

Printed in the United States of America by BookPrintingRevolution.com
First Printing: 2010

Jabberwocky Books
212 3rd Ave N
Suite 290
Minneapolis, MN 55401
www.jabberwocky-books.com

To order, visit www.LiveHappilyEverActive.com or call 1-800-797-4314. Reseller discounts available.

Photography by Michael Haug
Illustrations by Maria Franco

Cover and interior design by Erin Gibbons, The Designory (www.the-designory.com)

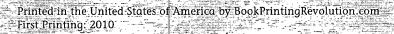